Complete Distributor's Guide
For TLC

Become A Better Independent Distributor

 # Life Changing Reps

Get Healthy & Help Others Get Healthy!

Terrell & Carol Barnes
Life Changing Reps

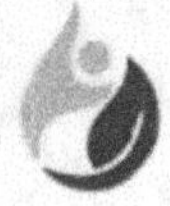

STRATEGIES FOR RESIDUAL INCOME

Welcome to TLC as an independent distributor!
Many families around the world are grateful for your help
within the health field.

We would like to share some techniques for you to build
your new business quickly. Hopefully you'll use these
strategies to bring-in some extra income and create a great
source for some residual income.

Your Life Changing Starts Now!

Introduction

I started my life of changes towards late summer of 2019 after my 42nd birthday. During the previous year I was diagnosed with type-2 diabetes, high blood pressure, and high cholesterol. I had many years of extreme substance abuse such as smoking, drinking, and eating all kinds of unhealthy foods. I was starting to feel numbness at the tips of my fingers as I awake most mornings after a night of heavy drinking. My right big toe was feeling numb at times as well. I was starting to feel sluggish throughout the first half of my days and didn't have the same strength I had while working my physical job.

Then I started to get random chest pains. Although it was only happening once-in-awhile, I had a feeling something was wrong. I went through a few years of depression after the deaths of a few relatives. First it was my grandmother, then my grandfather, then my son, my father-in-law, my cousin, my uncle, my aunt, and a few close friends. It was devastating and I turned to abusing toxic substances to calm my pain while I dealt with the stress. Not knowing that I was putting extreme stress on my body, I tried my best to cover my pain and hide my issues.

My wife who advanced in her health career was constantly on my back about going to the doctors to get checked, but just like most men, I brushed her advice off to the side. One day while working I had crucial chest pains and I tried my best to ignore it. I took a Bayer Asprin and waited for the pain to go away, but that time was different from others. Although I still didn't go right to the doctors, I still made an appointment which was a couple weeks later. After I got checked and was told that i was having minor heart attacks, had type-2 diabetes, a high A1C level, and numbers above 1200. We thought it was a miracle that I didn't pass out somewhere and found dead.

My ignorance almost caused my demise because I wasn't taking care of my body the way I should've been doing. I was developing spots all over my body and my skin wasn't looking clear as it was years previously. I lost most of my relatives due to diabetes, cancers, and other illnesses & diseases that could've been treated or stabilized. I was at my lowest point of life and I needed to make a change right away. So I started to cut down my smoking, drinking, and bad eating habits. I started working-out and lost 25 lbs. but still didn't feel quite good. It wasn't until I stopped eating the bad foods and putting the toxic things into my body when I noticed a tremendous change.

My drinking & smoking habits came to an end. I detoxed my body and started eating healthier food. The herbs, the vegetables, fruits, and natural supplements I started to digest made me feel better and greater than I've been in years. Although I was starting to go bald, I decided to shave my hair completely while my beard started to fill in. I finally had the feeling of hope once again. My attitude got better, I no longer had mood swings, and my decision making was better.

I began meditating as my vision for life got clearer. For years, I was running my own delivery service but that wasn't my passion. Of course, my wife noticed the changes I was making and she was finally starting to be at-ease with pounding me about my health. I started to become more conscious of human behavior and wanted to help make a change in other people's lives. I started helping people get jobs and making more money but I knew that wasn't enough for saving lives. We all know money can help people with their livelihood, buy the things they need and want, but money can't buy time and none of us can ever get time back.

After waiting patiently for my answer of what I needed to do throughout the rest of my life, I got an unexpected offer from my wife & her health partners. I was introduced to TLC, Total Life Changes and it was the perfect time. I was aware of the United States pandemic that was approaching, I was still upset about the relatives I lost due to health issues, and I already had a passion for helping people. So this was perfect for me to get involved. My wife was doing well and

I've seen her accomplish many things dealing with health. Once I began using the products from TLC and other recommended products, I started feeling better than ever.

When the Coronavirus pandemic took a major toll in our communities, I decided to go full stride. Not only did I help people make more money, but I helped them build-up their immune system and get healthier. That's when my blessings started to pour-in from different directions. I literally was in a position to start a new business which was in the health field. At that time, I was delivering medical supplies and specimens to hospitals and residents. But I was now able to turn down work & jobs that didn't fit into my new way of living. I started to meet and became friends with well respected people who were very intelligent in social behavior. Most-of-all, I was able to stay alive and be here for my beautiful family.

Now my wife and I are helping thousands of families all around this country get healthier & live longer. We wanted to provide this information for independent distributors as well as people who just want to make a change in their lives. We provided basic details about the best medicinal plants and herbs currently available to help strengthen our immune system. We hope all readers enjoy this short info book with lots of helpful insight for building your distributor business while learning about the best herbs, plants, and supplements for our bodies.

CHAPTER 1

We would like to share some basic modern techniques for building your business using the top social platforms. All the platforms we mention have been studied and tested over the past year with some of the top distributors, marketing experts, and ecomm specialists. Just to give an example, my wife/partner and I got over 7.8K likes, hits, and shares within the first week using these same methods and platforms.

We also got ranked on the top of Google search with only using one plain & simple ad. We didn't even have a good sales pitch at that time. My wife who's been in the health field much longer than me, got the TLC G5 ranking and helped over 1,000 families with their health issues in a short time period. When I partnered with her, we got on a faster pace of building our health business. We both have a passion for helping people so we decided to help our TLC family & other distributors reach a goal of life changing success.

Our health and immune system have been compromised by years of bad eating habits. Heart disease, cancers, diabetes, and many other illnesses fueled the fire for viruses and caused quicker deaths with people all around the world. Many vaccines and medications only stabilized most of the problems, but more problems developed due to the side effects. Those effects lead to taking more meds and getting more vaccines. It's a cycle that just keeps going on & on until the person eventually dies. Fortunately there are great opportunities to make the necessary changes needed to reverse most of these problems. By detoxing, strengthening our immune system, having better food intake, and helping others do the same, will change the lives of many people.

   You can also put yourself in a good financial position by distributing and selling products to help people get healthier. Anyone with an internet connection can search for wholesalers that sell in light bulk to small businesses, independent contractors, and affiliates. There's also multi-million dollar companies who give individuals the opportunity to join their company whereas they can get a discount on products for a better profit margin.

   Nature is the world's largest and most eclectic pharmacy. There's literally millions of species at our disposal that we can plant, cultivate, harvest, and use in our everyday lives. But most people remain uninitiated into the highly powerful realm of natural remedies that nature offers to us. Most people in our generation grew up disconnected from nature. Fortunately it is never too late for us to discover all the endless sources of natural remedies that are hidden all throughout the planet. Natural remedies can be grown almost anywhere. From large pieces of land, to small patches of ground, to flower pots, to small jars. Healing plants of all kinds and varieties can be bought at brick-&-mortar shops, online stores, or grown in your own garden.

Having a great love for life and healing yourself and/or others will give you a huge advantage during this day of age. I've compiled the best medicinal plants, herbs, vegetables, fruits, and supplements for anyone to grow in their own personal garden or purchase. I've also gathered great information for people who are affiliates or distributors to make more money.

From vegetables that help fight cancer and help prevent viruses and colds, to herbs that treat indigestion, skin conditions and anxiety, there is a healing plant and/or supplement discussed in this book. Most of these medicinal plants can be dried, powdered, made into teas, tinctures, soups, balms, soaps, syrups and salves. I'm sure you will find what you're looking for and what is best for you while on your journey to better health and helping others get healthier.

I want to dig right into some helpful information for you to quickly read, digest and put to use. For starters, if you are not making more than $500 hundred dollars per month, this might be the best info and investment you made for a TLC newbie. If you've already been making sales and building your team and business, it's time to boost your sales and pump up some nice passive income. I'm sure you know by now that TLC is rapidly growing and the competition is getting baffling. Let us help you crush it and jump over your competitors.

Now everyone involved in TLC is not doing it to help others. Many people joined the company for their own financial reasons. That's ok and entirely up to them and their personal goals. To get ahead of them, you will have to get passionate and extend a helping hand. Rather it be health advice, giving out samples, sharing helpful information, or just making friends in the health field, it'll be a good move to build an organic list of customers. A lot of people use word of mouth and social sites to do this but they do not use those platforms for business or have business accounts with them.

All TLC members get the same site pages to share and this could be quite boring for the experienced seller. Plus, if you are not binary qualified, you could be missing out on the extra payouts from your right & left downlines. But, if you're not binary qualified, don't worry, you can still make great profits as an independent distributor. Let's go over some ways to build your business and start your nice stream of

residual income in this billion dollar per year health industry.
I'm going to go through an easy step by step process that
you can arrange any way you'll like. No need for a complete
business plan yet.

First thing I would recommend is making a list of all your
family members, relatives, friends and neighbors that you
know who may have a health issue or might want to get
healthier. From that list, break it down into two categories.
Category 1 should be everyone you think who might need
your help with their health issue(s). The other category
should be everyone who you think might want to make some
extra money by helping people with their health.

Now you should create a pitch for the people on your list.
Do not be salesy or try to force your pitch. Instead, hook
everyone with the same line. Take a moment to pitch your
line to yourself. Look into a mirror and recite your pitch until
you can remember all the key details. Don't try to memorize
your complete pitch. It will be best if you can add a little bit of
freestyling to your lines so you don't come off like your
pushing for a sale.

Then make a copy of your pitch on a piece of plain white
copy paper, a file on your phone, or onto a file in your laptop
or desktop. You should have just one for each category. Edit
your copy and make sure it's the way you want to represent
yourself as being helpful. After you're done, create a master

pitch that'll go with the keys lines for both categories. This separate pitch will be like a pre-hype to introduce yourself as a "life changer" to everyone on both of your lists as well as people you might meet along the way, and people from your list who might share your pitch with others.

After you are done with your pitch, make some copies into fliers to give out. I would recommend getting black & white copies made on plain white copy paper or black & white copies on white glossy paper. You should start with 250 sheets. If you want to get the max amount of fliers, you should get four fliers printed on each page. This would give you smaller copies with 1,000 fliers instead of 250 full page fliers. Keep at least 50 fliers with you when you commute and travel. Then start handing some of your fliers out everyday for the next 30 days.

Now with your pitch from your two categories, you should start posting your copy on whatever social platforms you currently have. I highly recommend using platforms such as Facebook, Instagram, and Twitter for starters. If you want to get maximum exposure, I would suggest for you to start your own YouTube channel. Using the internet to advertise is the best way to run your new business or any modern business. For one, you could reach a lot more people without needing to travel. This would save you a tremendous amount of time and fuel. Secondly, you can actually get your flier in front of thousands of people in the health niche with only $10 - $20 right from your home, within just one hour or less.

Let's look into each one of these social platforms that I recommend. First we're going to start with the Facebook platform. Now Facebook has many rules you'll have to agree to in order to place ads on their website. Sure you can place a free post of your pitch or flier on your timeline, but you will not reach many prospects using that method. For one, Facebook only allows each person to have a max of 5,000 friends per account.

Secondly, you would have to depend on likes & shares just to get some good momentum. It would be a good idea to set up a Facebook Business page. With a facebook Business page, you'll get more tools for your post and all the tools & features are free to use. You'll only have to pay for the ads you want to send, and that's based on your selective amount of ad spend per day. This is far better than placing a post on your regular timeline, and you would be able to reach people who are interested in the health field that you don't have on your friend list or even know. This is the fastest way to grow your customer list and TLC business using the Facebook platform. You would be able to select your target audience, target area, as well as sub categories for the health field. Use this strategy for the next 30 days to get a good snowball effect and get ahead of other TLC distributors.

Using Instagram is different of course, but they have a good platform for building your business as well. You should create an Instagram business page as well. This will allow you to get more followers in a shorter time period than having a regular Instagram page. You should search for other people within the health field and start following them so your post could show up with a bigger audience. The more people you follow in the health field, the more followers you'll start to get and be able to advertise to them and whoever follows them.

I would recommend contacting some Instagram influencers to get maximum exposure. If you can find a good influencer, you can pay him or her an agreed amount of money per day to post your ad on their page for their followers to see. I suggest only paying influencers who have more than 100,000 followers. Use this strategy over the next 30 days to get further ahead of other TLC distributors.

The next social platform you should use is Twitter. I recommend using the Twitter platform only after using the Facebook and Instagram platform. Twitter is a good platform to use but far less effective than the other two platforms when building your TLC distributor business. You could take advantage of the Twitter platform like it's your personal business blog page. You should place tweets everyday about your TLC business. Even if your tweet doesn't have anything to do with your current ads, you still should place tweets about something dealing with TLC. I suggest only placing context ads and not video ads.

If you want to place video ads, I recommend using YouTube. First you'll have to create a YouTube channel. Creating a channel for your business is the best way to reach your audience using video content. Secondly, you'll have to use Google to set up your channel. Google is the owner of YouTube, so all your Google services will automatically get integrated with YouTube if you use the same email address.

After setting up your channel, you should place three videos within the first 3 days. This will give your video a way to get into the YouTube search so others can see your video without you needing to place ads. Make sure you turn on your subscribe tool for your channel to get subscribers and always ask viewers to subscribe to your channel on every video you create. When you get 1K subscribers, you'll be able to pay for ads.

If you're just starting with TLC as an independent distributor, I will highly suggest using these methods to build your business at a faster pace. This will definitely put you ahead of other distributors. You will also have much more momentum within your first 30 days with TLC. If you've been with TLC for a while, and you're not making at least $1,000 per month with TLC, I will suggest you give these methods a try. If you're making good income with TLC already, you can use these platforms with your current strategies to get more customers and sales. You can teach these methods to your downline as well.

CHAPTER 2

In this chapter we want to break down the top health products and benefits. This will give you a better understanding of how the TLC products can help with improving people's body and immune system. We will also go through a complete list of natural remedies that you could apply and market with your business without needing any kind of certifications. The breakdown will give you more insight and help guide you as you apply the recommended methods.

Instant Iaso Tea*

The unique blend is intended to provide gentle colon cleansing and natural body detoxification. This may also help to bring your body into balance and absorb more nutrients. The Iaso Tea works synergistically with TLC's full line of health and wellness supplements.

Iaso Tea with Full Spectrum Hemp Extract*

All-natural detox & cleanse with full spectrum hemp extract. People can enjoy the same great benefits of the original Iaso Instant Detox Tea with the addition of 100mg agricultural hemp extract. The all-natural proprietary formula is equipped with three additional extracts and combined with 2 grams of Nutriose FM06 (non-GMO soluble dextrin fiber) with only ten calories per serving. Hemp oil has been widely recognized for its many benefits on our human health. It has grown in popularity among the medical community as a critical supplement for maintaining homeostasis. This tea cleanses the upper and lower intestines, improves blood flow, helps reduce inflammation, promotes regularity and a healthy digestive tract.

Alleviate Cream*

Alleviate is a powerful proprietary topical cream with 21 all-naturals plus full spectrum hemp oil extract with naturally occurring phytocannabinoids. This topical cream provides one of the easiest ways to take advantage of the hemp extract benefits and can be used to target specific areas of medicinal pain and discomfort. Soothes irritated skin and unclogs hair follicles, reduces inflammation of the skin, aides in soothing aches, pains, and sore muscles.

Harmony Drops*

Harmony Drops is a full spectrum hemp extract. Harmony Drops can be used most commonly to assist with pain, stress, anxiety, poor sleep, inflammation, and chronic pain due to the cannabinoids present. There may also be an increase in your exercise performance, lean muscle mass, and aid in weight loss. Boosts your immune system, improves energy levels, digestion, and balances hormone levels. It also aids with a variety of health conditions, including headaches, muscle, and nerve pain.

Nutra Burst*

Nutra Burst is a daily multi-vitamin supplement. The bonded mineral base works to detoxify your system while supplying essential elements to strengthen your body. The liquid formula delivers an active blend of enzymes and nutrients found nowhere else. This complex multi-vitamin blend contains 13 elements including Ginseng, Grape Seed Extract, Green Tea Extract and Kelp. The amino acid complex includes the eight essential amino acids as well as the proteinogenic amino acids such as L-Arginine, Aspartic Acid, Cystine, Glycine and Glutamic Acid. Nutra Burst is unmatched in its Phytonutrient Enzymes and Whole Food Greens blends such as the proprietary blend of 72 minerals, 10 Vitamins, 22 Phytonutrients, 19 Amino Acids, 13 Whole Food Greens, and 12 Herbs.

CompleX*

CompleX is an immune support science-driven nutritional supplement that delivers an all-natural combination of potent extracts to support the immune system. It is intended to weaken viral infections, speed recovery, and keep the immune system functioning at its peak performance.

NRG*

NRG is a supplement to increase vigor, improve mental clarity, burn fat and curb your appetite. This all-natural formula is designed to provide results without jitters or sudden burnout. This is made into a capsule for easy digestion.

BlossoMĖ*

BlossoME is a women's balance formula which acts like estrogen in the body, balancing your hormones, controlling cravings and improving the complexion of your skin. It can also help regulate your body, your immune system, and control inflammation. Some of the all-natural ingredients include Ganoderma Lucidum (red reishi mushroom), Black Cohosh and Maca Root, all of which have been used in traditional medicine for years. Maca Root and Black Cohosh are intended to not only help with menopause symptoms, but they also aid in improving your mood and energy levels.

Chaga*

Chaga is called the "King of Herbs". The 100% pure Siberia Chaga extract is an all-natural immune-boosting superfood known for its high content of melanin and superoxide dismutase which functions as a powerful antioxidant. Chaga contains numerous vitamins and minerals. It is also one of the densest sources of Vitamin B5 which supports adrenal glands and digestive organs. It benefits the nervous system, the immune system, helps prevent damage to cells and tissues, and it has anti-aging properties.

Gano*

Gano is ganoderma lucidum also known as Reishi, is a medicinal mushroom. It has been used in traditional chinese medicine for at least 5000 years. It is known in China as Ling Zhi, and is considered to be "The Mushroom of Immortality". Reishi is the most potent adaptogen available. Adaptogens are those herbs and other substances that increase the body's resistance to stress and help it overcome health challenges more quickly.

The pure concentrated full spectrum Reishi is 100% Organic and 100% Kosher. It has Ganoderic Acids B, D, F, H, K, Mf, R, S, T-0, Y, Ganoderma Diol, Alkaloids, Anti- Oxidants,

Protein, Lingzhi 8, and Plant Sterols.

Techui*

Techui is 100% refined spirulina powder and a nutritious form of alkaline food. It is rich in protein, vitamins, minerals, chlorophyll and other essential nutrients needed daily by the human body. Used by Aztecs centuries ago, spirulina became increasingly popular when used by NASA astronauts in the 1970's as part of their diet. Spirulina high protein, and low calorie count makes it a superfood providing excellent nutrients. It is a natural "algae" (cyanobacteria) powder that is incredibly high in protein and a good source of antioxidants, B-vitamins and other nutrients. Spirulina improves the activity of white blood cells, stimulates antibodies and increases the population of natural killer cells.

ProZ*

ProZ is a natural supplement designed to assist in restoring the ideal microbiome composition in the gut. The high-quality probiotics in ProZ are intended to increase the number of good bacteria while the prebiotic fibers feed only the good bacteria helping restore proper balance in the most complex system in the body. This advanced, all-natural prebiotic, probiotic, and enzyme blend provides a gentle detoxing effect, promoting weight loss and a healthy digestive system for higher nutrient absorption and energy utilization, leaving you feeling great and craving healthier foods. ProZ formula is also designed to help you naturally and effortlessly relax from your day, fall asleep faster, sleep more soundly, and feel great in the morning.

HSN*

HSN is a daily supplement that provides six essential vitamins and important minerals. In addition to these essential nutrients, the HSN Supplement contains branched-chain amino acids (BCAA). These amino acids help trigger protein synthesis. In combination, the increased protein synthesis and the key nutrients provides the foundation for healthier, more vibrant hair, nails, and skin.

Stem Sense*

Stem Sense is a derived complex of an all-natural dietary supplement that delivers potent anti-inflammatory support compounds to help relieve joint and muscle soreness due to exercise or aging. This extremely multifaceted proprietary blend is designed to activate Nerve Growth Factor (NGF), and encourage healthier brain cell communication through the re-growth of neurites. Stimulate the growth factors that activate the stem cells in your body and replace worn-out cells to increase mental and physical energy.

Resolution Drops*

Resolution Drops are designed for those who want to lose weight quickly and safely without having to sacrifice their daily routine. The formula helps reduce food cravings, and relieves nausea, bloating, gas, and indigestion. Also reduces the likelihood of return weight gain. It has powerful ingredients to ensure a vital nervous system, helps calm the mind and assists with anxiety, and aids in controlling food cravings for weight loss.

Life Drops*

Life Drops is formulated with vitamin B-12, which has one of the largest and most elaborate chemical structures of all the vitamins. B-12 is essential for normal blood cell formation and supports health, energy, and metabolism in the body. It is responsible for many enzymatic processes that lead to growth, development, and the function of cells. It's needed to form adenosine triphosphate (ATP), and aids the body in improving circulation, suppressing inflammation and converting food carbohydrates to glucose, which is the most easily used source of energy. It has deionized water, vegetable glycerin, potassium sorbate, & stevia.

Slim AM*

Slim AM is a unique, high quality formulation synergistically designed for overall cardiovascular wellness by utilizing a combination of antioxidant components and L-Arginine to maintain endothelial cell performance and increased Nitric Oxide (NO) production. L-Arginine also stimulates the release of human growth hormone, insulin, and other substances in the body. Nitric Oxide relaxes the blood vessels allowing blood to flow. L-Arginine promotes stimulation of nitric oxide which helps support blood flow, vascular functions and intramuscular circulation.

Slim PM*

Slim PM is a three-benefit dietary supplement, designed to assist in Leptin control so you can burn fat while you sleep. The formula promotes optimum wellness and utilizes a combination of antioxidants and L-Arginine to target cardiovascular health and endothelial cell cleansing. It stimulates the production of anti-aging mechanisms with a powerful combination of antioxidants that supports intramuscular circulation while you sleep.

Matrix*

Matrix is a 100% organic plant-based nutrition shake with a complete balance of protein, complex carbohydrates, omega-3 fatty acids, branched-chain amino acids, adaptogens, digestive enzymes, probiotics, and high-quality fiber. It aids in weight management and muscle recovery, supplies the nutrition of a meal without the extra calories, helps increase vitality, decrease sugar cravings, and strengthen the immune system.

Delgada Coffee*

Delgada is a premium Arabica instant coffee powered with the natural strength of the Ganoderma Lucidum (Red Reishi) mushroom. Delgada provides the body with key nutrients, controls appetite, and aids weight loss. With consistent use of Delgada coffee, it may help people look and feel slimmer.

Plants in alphabetical order

Agrimony

Flowering Plant - Soothes urinary tract disorders such as cystitis and irritable bladders. It's anti-inflammatory when you use the flowerheads and leaves. Growing conditions prefer full sun.

Alder Buckthorn

Shrub/Tree - Relieves constipation and stimulates colon. Part of the tree for use is the bark. Growing conditions prefer damp soil conditions, deciduous hedging shrub, grows to about 5 meters tall.

Aloe

Evergreen Succulent - Healing properties for skin conditions such as sunburn, eczema, psoriasis, wounds and dermatitis. It is used to soothe and skin and prevent wrinkles. Helps ease gastrointestinal disorders such as indigestion and aids elimination. The parts for use are the fleshy leaves and pulp.

Growing conditions prefer sunny positions with moderate water, but water sparingly in winter.

Angelica

Herb - Appetite stimulator that treats indigestion. Eases cramps and prevents flatulence. Anti-inflammatory and the parts for use are the roots. Growing conditions prefer damp soil. Grows 2 meters. Harvest root in Autumn.

Aniseed

Genus - Fruit, that helps cure respiratory congestion such as colds and flu. Used as a digestive aid to help with colic, bloating and gas. Helps to control nausea and vomiting. Reported to enhance libido. Parts for use are the seeds. Growing conditions are annual in warm climates.

Artichoke

Vegetables - Lowers cholesterol production and soothes irritable bowel syndrome. Treats indigestion and helps digest fats by enhancing liver function. Parts for use are the flowerheads, leaves, and roots. Growing conditions prefer full sun, fertile, and well-drained soil.

Bilberry

Fruit - High antioxidants contribute to eye health, lessening the effects of glaucoma. Anti-inflammatory and anti-aging properties. Reduce the effects of vascular problems such as varicose veins, water retention and painful periods. Parts for use are the berries. Growing conditions prefer acidic soil, large pots and full sun. Fruits in summer.

Black Cohosh

Flowering plant - Reduces menopausal symptoms and balances hormones. Regulates menstrual periods. Soothes inflammation, and helps with arthritis. Parts for use are the root. Growing conditions prefer light shade and moist soil. Harvest roots in Autumn.

Blackcurrant

Fruit - Rich source of GLA. Treats skin conditions such as eczema. Reduces PMS symptoms, hypertension and rheumatoid disorders. Reduces blood pressure and alleviates swollen glands. Parts for use are the root, leaves, and berries. Growing conditions are full sun, requiring high nitrogen levels in soil (so add extra organic matter). Prune back in Autumn.

Black Mustard Seed

Fruit - Improves circulation, and helps stiff muscles, joints and cold extremities. Reduces inflammation. Parts for use are the seeds. Growing conditions are annual and the plant prefers light soil and moderate sun. Harvest seed pods in late summer, and dry in cool places.

Brahmi

Succulent - Improves mental clarity, memory and concentration. Parts for use are the aerial leaves & stems. Growing conditions thrive in warmer temperatures and tropical climates.

Burdock

Flowering plant - Detoxifying, antibiotic, antiseptic and mild diuretic effects. Helps with the treatment of skin problems such as eczema, acne, boils and dermatitis. Parts for use are the leaves, fruit, roots and seeds. Growing conditions are simple to grow and harvest seeds in summer.

Caraway

Fruit - Used to aid digestion, ease pain, expel gas, soothe bloating, prevent reflux and relieve heartburn. Parts for use are the seeds. Growing conditions prefer full sun and free-draining soil.

Celery

Vegetable - Anti-inflammatory. Taken for gout, anxiety, arthritis, and to aid sleep. A good diuretic. Parts for use are the stem and seed. Growing conditions prefer full sun, lots of water, compost and mulch.

Centaury

Herb - Used as a tonic for the liver and gallbladder. Stimulates appetite. Relieves disorders of the upper digestive tract such as heartburn and indigestion. Parts for use are the aerial parts. Growing conditions prefer full sun, and grow with other wildflowers.

Chamomile

Flowering plant - Helps reduce the effects of a variety of ailments such as anxiety, poor sleep, indigestion, colic, sciatica and gout. Often brewed in tea to calm nerves and enhance sleep. Parts for use are the aerial parts. Growing conditions: likes partial sun and poor soil.

Chaste Tree

Shrub - Relieves PMS pain, reduces hormonal acne, helps regulate hormones during menstrual cycle. Relieves menopausal symptoms. Parts for use are the berries. Growing conditions prefer sun and do well in most soils.

Cherry

Shrub - Rich in vitamin A, B and C. High in calcium and magnesium. Good general immune system booster with anti-inflammatory effects. Parts for use are the berries. Growing conditions prefer two plants planted for pollination. Likes full sun and needs damp soil.

Chickweed

Flowering plant - Soothes sore and inflamed skin. Mild diuretic. Soothes rheumatism. Vitamin rich and great in salads although they're classified as weeds. Parts for use

are the leaves. Growing conditions thrive in most soils.
Blooms in late winter to spring.

Chicory

Flowering plant - Mild laxative and anti-inflammatory. Can
lower blood pressure and cholesterol levels. Parts for use
are the leaves and roots. Growing conditions like
well-drained alkaline soil. Needs deep soil for root
development. Roots are harvested in the second year.

Chili

Vegetable - Used as an antiseptic, analgesic, stimulant and
tonic. Reduces muscular aches and pains and prevents
gastrointestinal infection. Parts for use are the pepper fruits.
Growing conditions prefer dry soil and full sun. Can easily
grow in pots.

Cinnamon

Tree - This is a powdered spice that has some amazing
medicinal benefits. The bark can be used for athlete's foot,
indigestion, improve brain function, and help lower blood

glucose levels. Parts for use are the bark that falls under the genus cinnamomum.

Cinquefoil

Flowering plant - Anti-aging benefits for skin. Treats fever, diarrhea, toothaches and mouth ulcers. Parts for use are the leaves. Growing conditions prefer full sun. Invasive and fast-growing.

Cleavers

Herb - cleavers is a good diuretic, assisting with swollen lymph glands, and many irritations of the urinary tract such as cystitis. Softens skin when applied. Parts for use are the leaves and roots. Growing conditions are annual and prefers alkaline soil. Known as goosegrass.

Cranberry

Fruit - Used to treat cystitis and other urinary tract infections. Parts for use are the berries. Growing conditions prefer part sun, part shade and moist acidic soil. Can grow in pots.

Cucumber

Vegetable - Help lower blood sugar levels.
Anti-inflammatory. Help to rehydrate and soothe skin. Parts
for use are the fruiting body. Growing conditions prefer
humid environments. Needs space to grow, and regular
watering.

Cumin

Flowering plant - The cumin seeds can help with digestion,
cardiovascular disease, urinary disorders, and fever. The
seeds can be dried and used to flavor food. Parts for use are
the seeds.

Daisy

Flowering plant - Used to heal wounds such as cuts, bruises,
sores and stiff joints when made into a salve. Helps reduce
the impact of respiratory tract infections such as sinusitis and
bronchitis. Parts for use are the flowerheads and leaves.
Growing conditions prefer full sun to grow.

Dandelion

Flowering plant - Dandelion has excellent detoxifying and diuretic properties. It also possesses vitamins A, B, C and D as well as potassium and calcium. It has been used to treat high blood pressure, cleanse the liver and gallbladder and treat skin problems such as acne and eczema. Parts for use are the flowerheads, leaves and roots. Growing conditions can be in sun and shade. Does best in well-drained soil, but tolerates most soil types.

Dill

Herb - Calms digestive disorders such as cramping, bloating and colic. When chewed can alleviate bad breath. Parts for use are the leaves and seeds. Growing conditions are annual. Easy to grow from seed, and requires 2 weeks germination.

Dragon fruit

Fruit - is a superfruit loaded with antioxidants. It grows on the Hylocereus cactus and is native to southern Mexico and Central America. Dragon fruit goes by many names, including pitaya, pitahaya, and strawberry pear. You can also get the full spectrum of nutrients with the added convenience of powder form.

Echinacea

Flowering plant - Highly effective for cold and flu relief. Antibacterial properties that help wounds and other skin infections heal. Parts for use are the roots and flowerheads. Growing conditions prefer full sun, rich and sandy soil. Harvest roots in Autumn.

Elderberry

Fruit - Antiviral and anti-inflammatory properties. Helps treat coughs, sore throats, cold and flu symptoms. Can be made into and taken as a tincture or syrup. Parts for use are the berries. Growing conditions prefer full sun. Should sow seeds in rich soil. Simple to grow.

Elderflower

Shrub - Can be made into cordials or wines. Antiviral and anti-inflammatory properties. Helps treat coughs, sore throats, cold and flu symptoms. Parts for use are the fresh flowers. Growing conditions prefer full sun, but tolerates shade. Pick only fresh white flowers.

Eucalyptus

Tree - Antiseptic and decongestant properties. The leaves have been used to remedy chest infections such as pneumonia and bronchitis, relieve muscle and joint pain, and cold and flu symptoms. Parts for use are the leaves. Growing conditions are the hardy species of tree that tolerates full sun and hot temperatures. Prefers well-drained, fertile soil.

Evening Primrose

Fruit - Rich source of GLA which assists bone health and regulates metabolism. Helps reduce PMS symptoms. Mild blood pressure reducer and soothes eczema. Parts for use are the roots, leaves and seeds. Growing conditions prefer full sun and low-nutrient soil.

Eyebright

Herb - Reduces the impact of eye infections such as conjunctivitis, and can be made into an eye wash for its astringent and antibacterial qualities. Also said to be a good lung tonic. Parts for use are the aerial parts. Growing conditions are annual and prefers full sun and chalky soils. Harvest the leaves and flowers while the plant is still blooming.

Fennel

Fruit - Appetite-suppressant for weight loss. Relieves bloating, cramping, flatulence and all kinds of stomach upset including colic. Parts for use are the flowerheads and seeds. Growing conditions prefer full sun positions with low water. Drought tolerant and attracts wildlife.

Fenugreek

Herb - Digestive aid. Soothes intestinal passages, sometimes used to treat gastric ulcers. Reduces cholesterol and blood sugar levels. Parts for use are the seeds. Growing conditions are annual and require full sun, but need shelter. Seeds ripen in 4-5 months.

Feverfew

Flowering plant - Commonly used to treat migraines. Reduces the symptoms of fever. Parts for use are the

leaves. Growing conditions are drought-tolerant and prefer
full sun.

Fig

Fruit - Gentle laxative that's high in fiber. Soothes stomach
pains and cramping. Parts for use are the fruiting body.
Growing conditions prefer well-drained alkaline soil and full
sun. Fruit ripens in summer.

Fleabane

Flowering plant - Diuretic and astringent properties. Lowers
blood pressure and helps treat kidney and menstrual
problems. Also said to prevent the attack of insects such as
fleas. Parts for use are the leaves and flowers. Growing
conditions are annual and prefers sun and light soil.

Frankincense

Tree - It can be used as an analgesic, antidepressant and
sedative, in addition to being a powerful healing herb.
Frankincense is also a primary ingredient in stress-reducing
incenses. Has a spicy smell and can be inhaled, absorbed
through the skin, steeped into tea, or used as a supplement.

Garlic

Vegetable - Antiviral and cancer fighting properties. Helps combat colds, flu and bronchitis, and lowers cholesterol. Anti-fungal properties good for treating fungal skin diseases such as athlete's foot and ringworm. Parts for use are the bulb. Growing conditions can be grown in pots and prefers sun and damp soil. Bulbs are picked in Autumn.

Ginger

Rhizome plant - Prevents all kinds of nausea such as vertigo, morning sickness, and motion sickness. Anti-inflammatory and good for arthritic joints and pains. Parts for use are the root. Growing conditions prefer shade with warm and moist soil. Not frost tolerant, so keep indoors in winter.

Ginkgo

Tree - Enhances memory and concentration. Soothes vertigo, leg cramps, asthma and allergies. Parts for use are the leaves. Growing conditions are slow-growing, prefer full sun and well-drained soil. Leaves must be harvested in summer.

Goji Berries

Fruit - Superfood that is said to boost circulation, improve eyesight, lower cholesterol, protect the liver, enhance immune function and improve libido. Has high levels of vitamin C. Parts for use are the berries. Growing conditions prefer full sunlight and fertile soil, but can grow in almost any soil type.

Gotu Kola

Herb - Commonly taken as a tonic for skin problems such as acne and digestive disorders. Aids memory and concentration. Anti-inflammatory properties give relief to rheumatism, arthritis and poor circulation. Parts for use are the aerial parts. Growing conditions prefer full sun to part shade. Needs well-drained soil.

Honeysuckle

Flowering plant - Painkilling properties useful for soothing sore throats, headaches and arthritis. Used to cool down hot flashes, sunstroke and fever. Parts for use are the flowers and buds. Growing conditions, deciduous shrub that prefers shade. Needs support as it is a climbing plant.

Hops

Fruit - Gentle sedative great for inducing sleep and relaxation. Great for reducing anxiety and abdominal tension. Assists with menopausal symptoms. Parts for use are the flowers. Growing conditions prefer full sun. Requires support and distancing from other plants.

Horse Chestnut

Tree - Seeds are used to treat haemorrhoids and varicose veins. Helps to decrease the likelihood of developing deep-vein thrombosis, and decreases the swelling of the lower legs during flights. Parts for use are the seeds. Growing conditions grown from seeds or conkers. Collect chestnuts in Autumn.

Horseradish

Vegetable - Used to soothe aching joints and muscles when made into a balm. Also stimulates the digestive system and lessens the severity of colds and coughs by clearing the nasal passages. Parts for use are the root. Growing

conditions can grow in large containers. Harvest roots in
Autumn.

Juniper

Tree - Berries have diuretic and anti-inflammatory effects.
Used to treat urinary tract infections, rheumatism and good
for gently lowering blood pressure and blood sugar levels.
Parts for use are the ripe berries. Growing conditions prefer
full sun.

Kiwifruit

Fruit - High in vitamin C, E, magnesium and copper.
Beneficial for improved heart function, improving eye health
and improving the quality of skin and hair growth. Parts for
use are the fruiting body. Growing conditions prefer part sun
and shade. Needs well-drained rich soil. Both male and
female plants needed to pollinate for fruit.

Lady's Mantle

Flowering plant - Stops external bleeding and encourages
blood-clotting when applied as a balm. The tea is effective in
preventing excessive menstrual bleeding and diarrhea. Parts

for use are the dried leaves and flowering stems. Growing conditions prefer dappled sunlight.

Lavender

Flowering plant - Wide range of calming effects, assisting in the relaxation of muscles, reduction of anxiety and enhancement of sleep. Eases irritability and aids digestion. Also helps with minor skin irritations. Parts for use are the flowers. Growing conditions prefer poor soil and full sun. Good to grow in pots. Harvest flowers in mid to late summer for drying.

Lemon

Fruit - High in vitamin C. Antibacterial and astringent properties. Used to reduce acne and brighten skin. Essential oil used to soothe fatigue and insomnia. Parts for use are the fruiting body. Growing conditions are all year-round, preferring part sun and shade with well-drained soil. Can grow in pots or in the ground. Needs to be fertilized in the growing season and watered in summer.

Lemon Balm

Herb - Used to soothe nervous tension, relieve anxiety and enhance sleep. Also effective in preventing the growth of herpes. Parts for use are the leaves. Growing conditions are very adaptable and grow in almost any soil. Fast growing and self-seeding. Requires constant pruning.

Licorice

Herb - Anti-inflammatory and anti-allergenic properties. Helps soothe coughs, sore throats and bronchitis. Prevent and cure gastric ulcers, and protect the liver. Parts for use are the root. Growing conditions prefer the sun and need a lot of depth for root growth. Roots are harvested from 3 to 4 year old plants.

Lime/Linden

Tree - Calms nervous disorders such as restlessness, anxiety and irritation. Good for treating colds and flu and lowers blood pressure. Parts for use are the buds and flowers. Growing conditions prefer cool climates in sunny positions. Needs moist soil.

Marigold

Flowering plant - Antiseptic and anti-inflammatory properties. Treats minor burns, insect bites, acne, cuts and abrasions, rashes and varicose veins. Parts for use are the flowerheads. Growing conditions prefer full sun. Easy to grow in containers.

Marijuana (Cannabis)

Shrub - Has potent psychoactive properties. Marijuana has been used to successfully treat and/or cure conditions such as glaucoma, high blood pressure, arthritis, depression, anxiety, HIV, cancer, multiple sclerosis, cerebral palsy and various other illnesses and disorders. It has potent sedative, anti-inflammatory and analgesic properties. Parts for use are the flowering tops of female plants. Growing conditions are annual. Requires rich, well-drained soil and full sun. Prefers slightly acidic soil.

Meadowsweet

Herb - Treats stomach disorders such as gastritis, indigestion and heartburn. Helps reduce severity of headaches, as well as inflammation of the joints. Parts for

use are the flowerheads. Growing conditions prefer damp
soil and full sun.

Milk Thistle

Fruit - Helps diminish headaches and digestive problems.
Popular "hangover cure". Helps treat and prevent hepatitis.
Parts for use are the seeds. Growing conditions prefer full
sun.

Mint

Plant - Medical herb that can help with stomach aches, chest
pain, poor digestion, fever, hiccups, ear aches and sinuses.
Can be used as a culinary herb and for medicine. Growing
conditions prefer wet and moist soils.

Motherwort

Flowering plant - Helps cure and ease the symptoms of
premenstrual syndrome, reducing swelling, anxiety and
irritability. Also used as a heart tonic. Parts for use are the
flowering stems. Growing conditions prefer part sun and part
shade. Easily grows from seed in poor soil.

Mugwort

Herb - Used as a liver tonic and also as an energy stimulant. Helps reduce anxiety, insomnia and depression. This herb has also been used for stomach problems such as cramps, colic and constipation. Parts for use are the leaves. Growing conditions prefer full sun and well-drained soil.

Mullein

Flowering plant - Expectorant and decongestant. Reduces mucus, soothes inflammation and aids in wound healing. Parts for use are the aerial parts. Growing conditions prefer full sun. Likes well-drained soil.

Neem

Tree - Anti-fungal, antibacterial and antiviral properties. Used to protect the liver, aid digestion and heal skin diseases. Also effectively kills lice. Parts for use are the leaves and seeds. Growing conditions grow in most soil types and prefer hot climates and well-drained soil.

Nettle

Flowering plant - High in vitamins, minerals and chlorophyll. Nettle leaves are commonly used to boost the immune system, reduce the pain of arthritis and joint swelling. They can also be used to treat dandruff and improve the health of hair. Parts for use are the leaves and roots. Growing conditions prefer nitrogen-rich soil. Harvest roots in Autumn.

Nutmeg

Tree - Helps to relieve muscle spasms, stimulate blood flow and prevent vomiting. Parts for use are the seed kernel. Growing conditions are from the Evergreen tree and it likes rich, deep soil in a sunny position.

Papaya

Fruit tree - Heals wounds and repairs skin. Reduces inflammation and also used to reduce the effects of skin conditions such as ringworm, psoriasis and carbuncles. Parts for use are the fruiting body. Growing conditions requires lots of sunlight and good quality soil. Requires frequent watering and a frost-free environment.

Parsley

Herb - High in vitamin A, B and C, protein, iron, potassium and magnesium. Anti-inflammatory and diuretic properties. Relieves flatulence, anemia and improves iron intake. Parts for use are the leaves, root and stems. Growing conditions prefer sunny positions. Easy to grow and can be grown in pots.

Passionflower

Flowering plant - Calming, sedative effects that soothe anxiety, tension, restlessness and sleep problems. Also aids in reducing stomach disorders. Parts for use are the flowerheads. Growing conditions prefer poor soil in a sunny position. Must be grown in a greenhouse in colder climates.

Pine

Tree - Decongestant, antiseptic properties. Commonly used as cough and cold remedies. Can also be used as a deodorant if made into a spray. Parts used: Pine needles. Growing conditions: Evergreen conifer that prefers full sun and acidic soil.

Plantain

Herb - Very effective remedy for insect bites. A natural source of antihistamine. Can also be used as a decongestant and expectorant. Parts for use are the leaves. Growing conditions are fast-growing and prefer full sun. Leaves can be used at any time. Can be used in teas or made into tinctures.

Psyllium

Fruit - Reduce bloating and swelling. Lowers levels of cholesterol and helps combat heart disease. Also helps to lower blood sugar levels and reduces the risk of colon cancer. Parts for use are the seeds/husks. Growing conditions are annual and need full sun. Seeds can be sown in late spring.

Purslane

Vegetable - Good source of vitamin E and omega-3. Used to treat gastric and liver ailments as well as arthritis. Parts for use are the leaves. Growing conditions prefer full sun and dry soil. Fast growing and not frost tolerant.

Red Clover

Flowering plant - High in isoflavones and phytoestrogenic compounds which is said to assist in menopause and PMS syndromes such as flushes, cramping and sweating. Parts for use are the flowerheads. Growing conditions prefer loamy soil and is easy to grow.

Red Raspberry

Fruit - Assisting in lightening heavy periods and helps to combat a variety of menopausal symptoms. Parts for use are leaves and the fruit which is rich in antioxidants. Growing conditions prefer partial sun to shade. Needs moisture-retentive soil and protection from birds.

Rose Geranium

Flowering plant - Soothes acne eczema. Antiseptic and anti-inflammatory properties. Used to also treat nausea, poor circulation and tonsillitis. Parts for use are the fresh leaves. Growing conditions from the Evergreen shrub that can be grown indoors. Water sparingly.

Rosehips

Fruit - Rich source of vitamin A, C, B vitamins and K. Commonly used to make cough syrup. Parts for use are the berries. Growing conditions prefer damp and heavy soil conditions.

Rosemary

Herb - Versatile herb that can be used in cooking and to relax the digestive tract. Also used to improve concentration, memory, reduce anxiety and mild depression. Additionally used to treat dandruff. Parts for use are the leaves. Growing conditions need full sun to grow. Thrives in most soils and must be pruned in spring.

Saffron

Herb - Powerful spice high in antioxidants that was used to treat stomach upsets, bubonic plague, and smallpox. Recent studies have indicated possible health benefits, including cancer-inhibiting properties, aiding in allergies, help combat depression, and promote a feeling of fullness, in terms of diet. Also improve mood, libido, and sexual functions.

Sage

Herb - Treats colds, coughs, tonsillitis, sore throats, inflamed gums and mouth ulcers. Also used as a memory enhancer, diuretic and digestive aid. Commonly used in flavouring cooked meats. Parts for use are the leaves. Growing conditions prefer full sun and dry soil.

Self-Heal

Flowering plant - Excellent plant for first aid, calming bites, burns, bruises, ulcers and cold sores when made into a salve. Antiviral properties that assist with reducing the effects of throat infections and inflamed gums. Parts for use are the flowering stems. Growing conditions prefer groundcover and alongside wildflowers. Tends to be invasive. Cut flowering stems in Summer.

Skullcap

Herb - Reduces the impact of anxiety, neuralgia, insomnia, tension and other nervous system disorders. Natural tranquilizing and antispasmodic effects. Parts for use are the aerial parts. Growing conditions prefer full sun and moisture-retentive soil. Harvest leaves in early Summer.

Slippery Elm

Tree - Recommended for digestive disorders such as constipation, colitis and ulcers as it soothes the gastrointestinal tract. Also used to soothe burns and skin irritations. Parts for use are the bark. Growing conditions require full sun to grow and prefers moist soil.

Soursop

Fruit - High in antioxidant compounds, including alkaloids, and flavonoid. Help stabilize blood sugar levels, reduce inflammation, fight bacteria, and help kill cancer cells. Parts for use are the fruit.

Spruce

Tree - Antimicrobial properties that prevent the growth of bacteria. Treats wounds, blemishes, bed sores, ulcers and other skin infections. Also makes a soothing inhalant for colds and flu. Parts for use are the resin and needles. Growing conditions like damp, acidic oil. Possible to grow in pots.

St. John's Wort

Flowering plant - Natural antidepressant. Used to treat mild to moderate depression, anxiety, seasonal affective disorder (SAD), insomnia, nervous tension and hysteria. Anti-viral and anti-inflammatory properties. Also treats cuts, bruises, inflamed skin and helps reduce the effects of herpes and hepatitis. Tends to conflict with prescribed birth control pills and antidepressants. Parts for use are the flowerheads. Growing conditions prefer a sunny position. Flowers in summer and self-seeds.

Tea Tree Oil

Tree - Possesses antiseptic, antibacterial, antiviral and antifungal properties. Excellent for treating skin problems and infection such as acne, ringworm, boils, athlete's foot, insect bites, cystitis, sore throats, thrush and other skin conditions. Like most medicinal plants, it can be infused, made into a cream or essential oil. Parts for use are the leaves. Growing conditions prefer sunny positions and lots of water.

Thuja

Tree - Used to treat the papilloma virus (responsible for creating warts). Also used to soothe sore muscles, neuralgia and rheumatic pains, as well as stimulating menstruation. Parts for use are the leaves and branches. Growing conditions prefer moist and deep soil. Prefers a sheltered site in full sun. Fairly easy to grow.

Turmeric

Rhizome vegetable - Anti-inflammatory, antioxidant and antibacterial properties. Used in India as a tonic for disorders of the liver and to heal wounds. Also used to treat arthritis, allergies, skin conditions such as psoriasis and high cholesterol. Parts for use are the root and rhizome. Growing conditions prefer light shade. Possible to grow in pots, but must be kept dry in winter.

Thyme

Herb - Antiseptic and expectorant properties. Helps to loosen phlegm from colds and flu. Soothe infected skin and aching muscles. Parts for use are the aerial parts. Growing conditions prefer gritty, well-drained soil in a sunny position.

Tulsi (Holy Basil)

Herb - Antispasmodic, analgesic, adaptogenic and anti-inflammatory properties. Lowers blood sugar levels, blood pressure and reduces fever. Often grown around temples in India and is revered as the herb sacred to goddess Lakshmi. Parts for use are the aerial parts.

Uva-Ursi

Shrub - Used to treat urinary tract infections such as cystitis. Leaves are used in tonics for the bladder and kidneys. Parts for use are the leaves. Growing conditions are the Evergreen shrub. Prefers damp and acidic soil. Leaves must be harvested in early Autumn.

Valerian

Herb - Natural tranquilizing properties that assist in sleeping and preventing insomnia. Also used as a sedative to calm anxiety, irritability and stress. Parts for use are the root. Growing conditions prefer partial sun and shade. Harvest 2 year old roots in Autumn.

Vervain

Flowering plant - Beneficial for a large number of ills including chronic fatigue, digestive problems, insomnia, depression, hot flushes, coughs and headaches. Useful for relaxing the muscles and soothing nerves. Also treats inflamed skin. Parts for use are the aerial parts. Growing conditions prefer lime soil.

Viola

Flowering plant - Anti-inflammatory properties that soothe eczema, acne, and other skin issues. Also serves as a diuretic, helping with various urinary disorders and cystitis. Can be taken as a decongestant for colds and flu. Parts for use are the flowers. Growing conditions are annual and prefer partial shade.

Watercress

Vegetable - Rich in vitamin A, B, C, E and minerals such as iodine, iron and phosphorus. Also contains cancer-fighting properties called PEITCs and sulforaphane which encourage cancerous cells to self-destruct, and builds natural defense against carcinogens. Used to treat arthritis, and can be made into a tonic for the skin and eyes. Promotes general health. Parts for use are the aerial parts. Growing conditions prefer boggy soil or shallow trenches and light shade.

Wheatgrass

Vegetable - Vitamin-rich and excellent for improving digestion. Used to treat diseases of the colon. Parts for use are the aerial parts. Growing conditions are annual and prefer rich, well-drained soil in a sunny position.

Willow Bark

Tree - Natural painkiller used in aspirin. Relieves inflammatory conditions such as rheumatism, osteoarthritis and back pain. Also used for menstrual pain, headaches, sport injuries and fever. Parts for use are the bark. Growing conditions prefer wet to damp soil and a sunny position.

Witch Hazel

Tree - Used for everyday ailments such as sprains, burns, bruises, blemishes, boils and other skin irritations. Also contracts the swelling of varicose veins and can soothe sore throats and laryngitis. Parts for use are the leaves. Growing conditions prefer damp soil and a sunny position.

Woodruff

Flowering plant - Used as a tonic to enhance liver function. Soothes arthritis. Acts as a mild sedative, helping with anxiety, restlessness and sleeping problems. Parts for use are the flowers. Growing conditions prefer groundcover, moist soil and shade. Fast-growing and tends to be invasive if not taken care of.

Wormwood

Herb - Used as a tonic to improve liver and gallbladder functioning. Also increases the production of bile and stomach acid easing digestion and preventing bloating and gas. Serves as an excellent insect repellent. Parts for use are the leaves and flowerheads. Growing conditions prefer full sun and poor well-drained soil.

Yarrow

Flowering plant - A versatile plant that can be used to treat coughs, colds, aid digestion, stop diarrhea, stop bleeding, heal bruises and rashes, and prevent headaches. Parts for use are the flowers and leaves. Growing conditions prefer a sunny position.

End Of List

It's important for you to keep in mind that not all of these medicinal fruits, vegetables, trees and herbs are possible to grow in your area of the world. Some could be illegal, and may also be harmful for pregnant or nursing women. You should test your reaction to some of these plants before consuming or applying to your skin. Some of these medicinal plants may interfere with prescription drugs, so it may be best to consult a doctor first. Otherwise, these are some really powerful natural remedies and healing plants which you can benefit from. Visit our website for a full catalog of health & wellness products. [LifeChangingReps]

CHAPTER 3

Now let's talk about how you can take your business up another notch. Getting your own website would be the next phase for growing your distribution business and putting yourself in control of your own content and products. Doesn't matter if you use a free site builder or pay a webmaster to create your content, you would be able to add more products that TLC may not have. Plus if TLC runs out of stock, you will not have to keep your customers waiting on their products. Running out of stock isn't good when you have a product in high demand and your customer(s) is waiting much longer for their delivery.

Study these plants, herbs, and remedies mentioned in this book. This will give you great advantage when you can help almost anyone with almost any health issue(s) they may have. You can buy these plants & products at wholesale prices, then put your mark-up value on them as you resale for profits. At this time, no one is really doing this, or using these strategies, so you'll be much further ahead of others distributors. Just imagine being the person who can help a lot of people get healthier without needing to take medication or vaccines. Plus, being the person who can supply them with the proper remedy.

The demand for health products has exploded since the beginning of the Coronavirus pandemic. This is a great time to reach out to others who have interest in the health field and partner with them. Maybe your significant other, close relative, friend or another TLC distributor. Create a mutual agreement and start doing some marketing together. Start your own blog, blog page, or catalog and use the pitch from your list in the beginning to place posts every week. All you'll have to do is tweet your pitch according to the response you'll get from the people on your list. Try to answer all your replies and questions.

As you start to build your audience and your own platform, you should define your expertise. Your visitors need to know why you are credible, and why you are different from all the other distributors. You should highlight what sets you apart, but don't disparage your niche. TLC distributors who badmouth their competition appear gimmicky and overly sales-oriented. Draw attention to the elements of your narrative that may uniquely connect with people. Tell your health story and journey in a way that promotes relatability and know-how. By doing this you'll promote credibility and likability at the same time.

Developing a personality as an independent distributor for TLC will help you create great content to build the TLC brand as well as your own brand as a nutrient expert. When you infuse your own online space with your beliefs, experience, feelings, thoughts, and values, people will start to make opinions. Positive opinions are very good, but negative opinions are good too. The key to curating a personality is to not be boring while helping people with their health issues. Highlight the intense elements of your pitch content and draw out the parts of your pitch that will catch the eye of visitors.

There are no shortcuts here. Great content will be the best foundation for distributor success. Your content must be helpful and engaging. It must be honest and valuable as well as compelling. It needs to be as short as possible, without any extra fluff. If you skimp on this step, you will pay for it in the future. There's many distributors out here that's not making much money. In fact, most distributors are making far less per month than their weekly salary at their regular employment. It's imperative that you take a different approach if you want to see different results as an independent distributor.

The process may take a few days or weeks, so don't try to monetize right out the gates. If you don't pace yourself and put in the energy to build your list, brand, and personality, your brand will look flimsy and too salesy. Focus on building an audience that connects to you, your brand, and TLC on an emotional, authentic level. As a member of TLC, don't forget to promote connections throughout your community. This means honestly participating in forums relating to health, not just posting links.

Having real conversations, getting to know people, and getting involved in helping them get healthier will be highly recommended. Just because your sales platform is internet-bound doesn't mean that person-to-person business tactics don't work. Extend a virtual meeting every week to people in your downline and people you might want to work with in the future. Do guest posts on blogs. Attend TLC conferences in person. All of these actions, online or offline, add to your brand and distributing business.

Keeping in contact with your customers is paramount to achieving success as a TLC Independent Distributor. Check in with your customers and ask how they're doing. Ask about what kind of health issues they have and what kind of remedies they prefer. Share good information that would be genuinely helpful to them. If the people on your contact list know that your content is more than just quick sales pitches, they will continue to open them and engage with your post, brand and products. If you're getting the kind of results you hope for right away don't worry. All the top distributors took a little time to build their success. So don't let your excitement fizzle out. As with many things in life, it's common for new business owners to put in a lot of effort up front but lose steam when they don't get the results they were hoping for quickly. Push through and remain consistent in your efforts to get the big, sustainable results.

   I would suggest you only promote the products you're passionate about. An important aspect of achieving success as a TLC distributor is promoting products you care about. Using this as a general rule of thumb will make sure that you bring authentic energy to your promotions, which will translate into credibility. Before you promote a product, it is a good idea to try it out first. You can buy the product, or you can reach out and get a sample for a review. Once you have the product, you can really invest in using it and documenting the results. This will provide good information for future content and will help you answer any questions potential customers might have.

Take pictures of your results for your own review. Create video content to post on the social media platforms you use, especially on your YouTube channel. Put links to the products in your detail description. If you can, give out samples of that same product in exchange for a review from the person you're giving the sample. Create bonuses and contests for the people on your list, and on your pages.

Give your visitors a chance to get or win a free product. Ask them to post a review about the product you gave them so you could build more credibility. The number one rule when it comes to promotion products is to approach your audience with respect. When you treat potential customers like real people with goals, fears, and hopes for better health, you will build trust with them. They will start to see you less as someone trying to sell them something and more as someone who is credible and wants the best for them.

In my opinion and my experience, Godaddy has the best website platforms for beginners and people who want to accelerate their business at a fast pace. Not only would you be able to promote the TLC products you like, you'll be able to build your own storefront and set your own prices. If you want to upsell your customers into something bigger and better, you can do that. This method would bring in more income for your business. It's like having a great salesperson on your team or downline that works for free. You can give your customers fresh selections of products and prices by varying your product promotions. Godaddy supplies robust and detailed reports to help you expand your service-offerings and drive sales.

If you'd like to earn generous commissions through referral sales from your website visitors you should check out their Affiliate Program. In addition to that, if you are looking for a way to help your team or downline manage all of their customers and clients, Godaddy has a dashboard with a ton of integrated tools. Unfortunately TLC customer service isn't as good as it should be, but Godaddy has great customer service and you'll be able to reach someone 24/7. They can help you at almost every stage of your journey. Whether it's for your inspirational videos, informative blog posts or friendly business guides, they will take your call.

Using these methods for your distributing business would help you get more momentum and grow faster than many other distributors. This would certainly put you ahead of others if you follow the recommended steps and stay consistent. Keep in mind that these methods and strategies are based on our opinions and may be different for each individual. For the most part, it will all depend on how you choose to build your business. If you want to add more strategies, I also recommend networking and attending some of the live TLC events.

   When you go to the live events you should have all your marketing material ready and in order. If you have any ideas that may help your business grow, you should add them at any time. One more helpful tool I suggest is getting your own business phone line. If you don't want to pay for a second phone service, you can get a business line feature from Grasshopper. They have an unique service whereas you'll get a business service added to your current phone line. You'll be able to have your own business voicemail and ringtone so you'll know when you're getting a business or personal incoming call.

   These methods will put you way ahead of other distributors within 30 days if you put it to use. We hope this information was helpful and that it'll help you get a better profit and ROI. If you use these methods, you should get more customers and sales. Our final advice is to be consistent with your marketing strategy.

For those who just want to get healthier, we hope you try one of these to help you with whatever issue it may concern. If you're currently taking any kind of medication, you should check with your doctor before consumption.

Best wishes and much success in your journey!!!

Success Stories

A guy by the name of Phillip Birchfield has been making moves within network marketing since he enrolled in Total Life Changes which he graduated to the rank of Global Director. His strong performance of ownership and running his family business has driven his success. In turn, he pushed his daughter Jacqueline to the top. Although she was a fan of the TLC products which her father had introduced her to, she didn't immediately get into the business.

She was drinking the Iaso Tea because it made her look and feel better. In fact, she lost two pant sizes and was very happy with her experience with the Iaso Tea. At first she was shy about telling people how the TLC products were helping her make the improvements she wanted to make. When she was considering selling the Iaso Tea, she said that she felt weird about the idea of selling it. Eventually she just couldn't deny her belief in the TLC line, and decided to join the TLC family with the greater opportunity it offered.

Jacqueline said her public speaking skills have improved dramatically, as well as her education in the health field. Over the past few years, her TLC family has been there by her side through the birth of her second child and her graduation from college. After she graduated, she was able to walk away from corporate America as a regional director at the age of 23. She was able to focus on TLC full time while being a stay-at-home mom. Jacqueline's short-term goal was to accept a $250K earner ring at the company's Dallas 2019 conference. Her longer term goal is to "take over" her hometown of Fort Wayne and help even more stay-at-home moms become financially independent.

Phillip is a resident of Fort Wayne, Indiana, who became part of the TLC model for success. He joined the company in May of 2014. He made $100,000 in income in his first year and now he leads a team of thousands of distributors and marketers. Like many of TLC's top earners, this isn't his first experience in the network marketing field. In fact, Phillip spent more than 20 years with various companies building hundreds of teams. But yet, he was never able to get over the hump with any of those companies. As hard as he worked in network marketing, he never built any residual wealth with any of them.

Having personally struggled with his weight, Phillip was shocked at the results when he sampled the Iaso Tea. He lost 2 lbs within the first day of trying it, and ultimately lost over 40 lbs. After he took a look at TLC's compensation plan, he called up his sponsor immediately. Phillip wanted to help a lot of people and make some money along the way. It became his mission to show people that network marketing is a level playing field. His mother Edna Ellis is a 6 figure earner with TLC, and a National Marketing Director. His daughter Jackie Birchfield is a Regional Marketing Director, and received her $50,000 earner ring in Atlanta.

It seems like TLC success ran in Birchfield's blood, but he would not have reached the rank of Global Marketing Director without his great personality and a strong work ethic. His activity on social media helped him spread the word of his accomplishments and he was able to make connections in some unexpected places.

He recognizes new potential team members when he meets them, and gives them the practical support they need to grow. He recently began mentoring a powerful Amish couple by the name of James and Rose Lengacher. He also helped them understand the compensation plan. They're now National Marketing Directors of TLC. The Amish team has grown exponentially, and he regularly supports their meetings and events. Phillip's radical success is a testament to the possibilities TLC offers to those with the passion and vision to pursue their dreams of success. He started from zero with TLC, and now he's able to give thousands of dollars to the local Boys and Girls Club every year.

Giovanna Munoz is a wife, commercial engineer and mother of 3 children. She knows the value of staying busy and working hard. But she was determined to improve her financial situation. Giovanna sought additional financial opportunities and learned about the compensation plans in the MLM industry, especially at TLC. Giovanna joined TLC in 2016. She was introduced by her successful mutual friend named Fermín Vera.

Fermín has been her guide in the process of change. When he presented TLC´s Compensation plan, she couldn't say no. Shy and introverted, Giovanna's said her biggest challenge was herself and she knew it was going to be hard work. Giovanna had to develop the skills and confidence she needed in order to succeed. She said her financial goals and getting out of debt was bigger than her fears and shyness. She earned $600 in her first month and now she's a National Director at TLC, generating more than $11,000.

She considers TLC her second family because everything in the company is about partnership, loyalty, and love. Since TLC has products that work, and an amazing compensation plan, many people have made the decision to join the company all over the world. Giovanna's family is also involved in the business. Her aunt has already generated more than $15,000 in one year and her husband earned $5,000 in only 4 months. Giovanna's favorite product is the

Iaso Tea. The tea has helped her with her digestion and helps eliminate fluid retention from her body.

She was even able to lose 7 lbs in five days. She said TLC is a blessing and the company allows you to have quality time with your family and with your business partners. Now she's able to travel with her husband as they discover the world together. They also were able to buy a new car and improve the education for their children. One of Giovanna's short-term goals was to impact more families with TLC opportunities and openings in new countries. Her long term goal was to position herself in all the continents of the world.

In 2012, at the age of 17, Jason Rodriguez was already taking his first shot at working in multi-level marketing. When that initial experience didn't work out, he ended up struggling through rough 12 hour days of employment. But Jason wanted more and was willing to take risks. Jason discovered TLC when his mother was invited by a family friend to a meeting. Once he accepted the TLC opportunity, his first 48 hours were very surprising. He managed to enroll two people to become binary qualified. By his ninth day in the business, he became a Director and made a very significant first week income. According to Jason, the keys to his success are dreaming big and having strong support from his family.

Within 18 months of being a TLC distributor, Jason achieved one of his most ambitious goals of becoming the company's youngest National Director. His current income often reaches five figures per month. Jason said NutraBurst, Iaso Tea, and Chaga are his favorite products because they help provide him with the energy he needs to build his expanding business. He's part of a movement called RichBefore30, which works with young people to help transform them into entrepreneurs. He plans to help five people to create a six-figure income and clear 10,000 team members overall. He also wants to create a youth movement in MLM.

Melaine Bernard's approach to building her TLC business was methodical and pragmatic. She relied on some of her past business experience to help. When it came time to publicize her line of work, a video on social media was enough to do the trick for her. After her video, everything came together very quickly for her. Within weeks, hundreds of people she didn't even know started to follow her on social media. It was the perfect way to get a conversation going about TLC products. Thanks to TLC, Melaine has obtained financial freedom and the freedom to use her time the way she likes. For a couple years, she traveled across Europe to meet her IBOs during the TLC Tour Connection which is an event she created. She describes them as incredible encounters filled with gratitude and strength.

Some of Melaine's success came from thinking of TLC as an extension of her family. Melaine has become a Global Director which is one of the highest ranks within TLC. She is the first Global Director in Europe. She intends to become a company Ambassador, significantly augmenting her already 5 figure monthly income, and by 2019, an Executive Ambassador, the top of the TLC pyramid.

Lenika & Gregg Scott, are partners and best friends. In 2013, Gregg & Lenika became leaders in building a sales force with TLC. They decided to join the direct sales company because it focused on making it possible for people all over the world to improve their health and make money while working from home. Their business has financially restored their lives and allowed them to live a debt free life. Within a few months of their distributing partnership with TLC, Lenika & Gregg and their team members were able to hit the 6 figure income margin in record breaking time. Together they are seeing incredible results by helping their team. Within one year of joining TLC, they were half million dollar earners and after two years, they received their $2 million check.

Today the Scott's portfolio continues to grow through their added companies, including their web design business which services others with personal branding, social media, and websites. Thanks to their work with TLC, in 2015, the couple achieved their goals of purchasing their dream home and living debt free.

Gregg & Lenika are Legacy Builders who are empowering communities to leave a Legacy. They help others tap into their full potential through empowerment, leadership skills, and building self-confidence. Their home based business empire has allowed them to travel the world. They often treat their family to numerous trips and vacations. After years of not being able to travel at all. They can now afford luxury items and a lifestyle they never could've imagined before.

Twiler Portis is a former corporate executive. Twiler partnered with her late husband Erwin Portis, to build distribution networks of over 350,000 people in the United States and 6 other Countries, to build an enterprise in the network marketing industry. They partnered with TLC and became one of America's most admired power couples. Through their partnership, thousands of business partners were able to quickly transform. Not only did they transform lives, but their bank accounts too.

Twiler joined other marketing moguls and in one short year, added more than 15K business partners within the TLC tiers. Twiler has been the source and secret weapon in the success of more than 20,000 network marketing businesses and distributors. Twiler set her sights on expanding her vision through her brand and to inspire people to use their life's worth to fuel their passion. She equipped individuals with tools and resources to turn their obstacles into opportunity.

She partnered with thousands of businesses to mentor, coach and train them, resulting in thousands of families receiving 5 & 6 figure incomes per month. Twiler has soared to the top of a lot of companies, reaching their top positions and breaking records. Her accomplishment has landed her on the cover of company magazines. She has been featured in national publications and television shows. Twiler's entrepreneurial spirit, and her passion for business has afforded her the unique opportunity to executive produce television shows, invest in business start-ups, and mentor small businesses. Her work brought her to large stages, taking her words globally. Even in the darkest of times, her strength has been an inspiration to many.

She's a champion in the health and wellness field. Twiler's online audience can be found working on business goals while focusing on living their healthiest lives. She's a mother to a teenage entrepreneur, fashion designer and musical artist. Twiler entered 2018 with one goal in mind, to recruit and mentor the next great crop of successful entrepreneurs.

With coaching and mentoring, Twiler is looking for the next success story.

Fermin and Belen were in a difficult financial situation with personal and family debts. They started searching for opportunities to get ahead so they could live happier. Luckily, in May 2015, their sponsor and TLC Ambassador, sent them information about TLC products & business opportunities and they were instantly hooked to multi-level marketing. TLC's sustainable compensation plan is one of the reasons they decided to join. They were also attracted to TLC's family environment because they love the idea of everyone sharing and supporting each other. While Fermin and Belen were excited to start their new business, they knew it was the opportunity to get them where they wanted to be.

At their first business seminar, they set up chairs, spread out tables with products, and displayed audiovisual materials, yet no one showed up. Fermin and Belen believe in TLC very much, so they didn't let that stop them. They continued to focus on their business and making it at TLC. Now, they have hundreds of people on their team. They have a lot of clients with weight loss and financial testimonies. Partnering with TLC, they didn't only helped themselves, but they've also helped many families change their lives.

Professional speaker, trainer, author, entrepreneur, and TLC Ambassador James Dentley knows a thing or two about distribution. As a successful entrepreneur for over 30 years, he has helped over 400,000 people throughout the world become high performers in their business and personal lives. TLC has been thrilled to have him as part of their growing team. James joined TLC in December 2013, at that same time, he was expanding his own company. He saw a vision and opportunity to help many people that were struggling with their health and it all just made sense.

He knew TLC products could help so many people. As a business strategist, and entrepreneur he knew that if it worked he would be very successful. His wife, Kara Dentley is a National Director with TLC and their two children are all in the business standing by the products. James has been a part of four companies in the last 25 years, but none of them compared to TLC. James has shared the stage with some of the best across the world. He has been in business for over 30 years and has trained over 400,000 people around the world to become successful in their professional and personal lives. Not only that, but he has also helped many companies to excel in the areas of training, profitability, communication, and leadership development.

Erika Delgado saw the numbers TLC was doing, so she took a leap of faith, left her stable job of eight years as a secretary with the National Army of Colombia, and joined TLC. Erika met TLC in June 2016 after watching a YouTube video. She started by using the Original Iaso Tea and Resolution dietary supplement. After seeing such amazing results with her health and her body, she made the decision to join the company and start her own business.

Her entire family thought she was crazy to resign but she was sure about the TLC opportunity and their products. Since joining TLC, Erika's life has changed so much that she has even involved her family in her vision. Her father is a Director with TLC and her mother and husband are both Executive Directors. Erika has not only experienced the positive physical benefits of losing weight with TLC, but she has also experienced incredible health benefits. With TLC amazing products, compensation plans, and outstanding leadership, Erika knew she was on the road to success.

TLC is continuously changing the lives of millions of people across the globe, and Erika is excited to be a part of the movement. Erika achieved Global Rank with TLC and is continuing to help many Life Changers on her team grow mentally, physically, and spiritually. Erika is extremely focused on the health and growth of her team. Erika is committed to expanding the growth of her organization. She had several events in Mexico during 2019. Her mission to help 1,000 families was accomplished quickly. She already has a team in several countries around the world. She has her sponsor, Global Director, Christian Prada, and TLC's leadership team to thank for continuously guiding her towards the path to true freedom.

Dominicano Julio Lama is a businessman, engineer, coach, leader and father. But in the TLC dictionary, there's only one word that adequately describes his contributions which is Ambassador. Lama became TLC's first male Latin American Ambassador, the second highest rank an Independent Distributor can reach under TLC's compensation model. That accomplishment reflects the vast organization Lama has stewarded, with over one hundred affiliates earning between $10,000 and $250,000 per year.

Latin America has rapidly become a cornerstone of TLC's global operations. Prior to joining TLC, Lama had already lived an interesting life by holding numerous postgraduate degrees. His intellectual curiosity and ambition stood to his credit when he began working with TLC in June of 2015. While considering network marketing a supplement to the income of his successful engineering career he knew he had the right products. Like many IBOs, Lama has a personal testimony with TLC products that has helped to fuel his passion to grow the company.

When he started TLC he weighed around 300 pounds. He specifically credits Iaso Tea, Resolution, Slim PM, Slim AM and Delgada slimming coffee with his improvement, and many people within his organization have similar success stories. Many of the benefits were clear to him. The first thing he likes to point out are the commitment and loyalty TLC has to each of its independent distributors, the quality of the products and its sustainable compensation plan.

As he continued to move up the ranks of the company, he also began to see how the success of his own organization has had a beneficial effect on his community. He genuinely believes TLC is bringing hope, health and financial freedom to those with an affinity for direct marketing. As a result of the success of many of his friends and team members, we're seeing money flowing into their communities in Latin America. Under Lama's watch, many in his organization have reached high ranks, including a number of National and Global Directors.

Jose Luna is TLC's new Global Director. Jose grew up in a small town in El Salvador in Central America, and is currently living in Long Island, New York. He joined TLC in February of 2016. He had the privilege to meet his sponsor, from a previous business venture. Jose knew the opportunity that he was ready to take would make a difference in many people's lives. He understood his sponsor's drive, his passion, and his work ethics which were a great match for TLC.

Jose's purpose for joining TLC is to leave a legacy for his family. Jose proclaims that Iaso Tea has made a big difference in his life. When he started drinking it on a regular basis, the changes in weight loss, skin, and overall health were incredible. It became part of his daily life. The NutraBurst is another one of his favorites. The energy and the abundance of nutrients, supplied him with all he needed. He reinstates that it's essential when daily intake is not met.

Jose is no stranger to the full lineup of health, wellness and beauty products. He tried them all and he loves the difference it's making to his health. Acknowledging others' results while using the products and the changes in their lives is exciting and inspirational to him. Many of his customers are having great results with the Iaso Tea. They are losing up to five pounds in five days just as a result of detoxifying their system. And the NutraBurst is very popular among mothers because it is a safe liquid multivitamin for everyone in their home, including their pets.

Jose Luna recognizes TLC as a truly amazing company. Grown from the basement of Founder and CEO Jack Fallon's in 1999 to a Top 100 Global Direct Selling Company. Working with TLC and the success behind their teamwork's proven results is inspirational to him. The long-term relationship with families is what motivates him to continue. His monthly income continues to increase and he's grateful to have had the opportunity to make 6 figures in a short amount of time while at TLC.

Jose indicates that TLC has provided a chance for self expression, team development, but most importantly, mirroring what a corporate family is. He states that the key difference TLC offers is the diversity and the support between everyone. Jose is aware that TLC is attracting a diverse demographic of entrepreneurs like himself, and he agrees it's the great products and amazing compensation plan that sets it apart. The extraordinary leadership is what pushed him to his short term goal of developing 50 National directors. His long term goal pertains to helping 1,000 families become debt-free within a three-year time frame with TLC.

A lot of people may have heard about the success of Dexter and Tonya Joyner-Scott in TLC, but nothing matters more to them than witnessing the success of many business partners that have joined forces within the last 18-24 months. It hasn't been an easy path to success for this married couple. They faced adversity, doubt and the loss of a 6 figure income before they restored their lives with network marketing.

Tonya has carried her fears and limited beliefs of her future for much of her life.

Those negative attitudes even caused her to become complacent for a while as she began to start a family. She kept trying to tell myself that being a stay-at-home-mommy was enough for her, but it really wasn't. She was dying inside because she was no longer living up to her fullest potential. Her husband was traveling around the world impacting the lives of children and teenagers.

He had studied with industry leading speakers and trainers like Les Brown and Paul Martinelli, but yet he found it harder to share all of these wonderful things he was experiencing with his wife because he knew she was struggling with self-doubt. Dexter was unfortunately laid off from his 6 figure income, just before leaving the country for a family vacation. It was during this time that the couple did some soul searching.

Some people may call it destiny, while others may consider it fate. But Dexter and Tonya felt it was more like divine intervention. It was that action that brought them to TLC. The fear they carried most often was the fear of failure. Not only the failure for them, but the failure of those that may be joining them as well. This was one of the reasons they sat on this opportunity for as long as we did. But losing a job changed everything. They knew they had to face their fears and do this together for their family and for others.

When they overcame that fear, they were so grateful to be a part of this amazing company. Now they have a multitude of people earning great income and advancing in rank month after month throughout our organization. Recently, one of their personally enrolled Directors purchased a luxury vehicle after her transmission blew in her previous car. It was because of her commissions with TLC that she was approved for her car loan. They have also been blessed to watch Regional Directors experience more time freedom since partnering with TLC. Another great example of how their leadership and team building has led to other people's success is through Executive Director Laura Bethea.

Laura is working toward the completion of her doctorate degree in Educational Leadership in Higher Learning from East Carolina University. She has been able to pay her tuition each semester as a result of her TLC commissions. Another example is that of Global Directors Darnell and Dr. Kimberly Edwards who paid off more than $30,000.00 in debt. These are just a few stories throughout Dexter and Tonya Joyner-Scott's organization of partners experiencing success with TLC. Everyone is finding joy in helping someone feel better, look better, sleep better, and be better.

Their mission is to help their distributing team move forward with intentions on changing people's lives for the better.

Success in the distributing industry all depends on the leadership as well as developing specific qualities to grow and sustain momentum in your team. Ana Cantera has been experiencing explosive growth. She's built a solid international business that led to her becoming the first IBO to achieve the rank of Ambassador with TLC in Latin America. Ana's team dedication to provide their new enrollments and customers with strong support defined their tremendous success.

Cantera has shown that there is no challenge or adversity that can stop her. Without any experience in the industry, she was able to reach one of the highest positions at TLC, with earnings over 7 figures in the past 3 years. She built organizations of more than 20,000 distributors around the world. She committed to help people achieve their health and wellness goals. She shares a vision for building residual income to foster their dreams.

Success in Network Marketing should not depend only on yourself. One of the biggest reasons many people don't achieve the results they want is because they don't care about the needs of their team. Building a business requires lots of time, effort, and patience. Working together as a team will help you achieve success quicker and easier. Ana was introduced to TLC by Executive Ambassador Stormy Wellington. Ana has quickly expanded TLCs vision in the Latin American market and she's determined to continue to impact families worldwide. TLC has amazing and innovative products, which covers multiple needs in society, ensuring a residual income for life. Ana works with an outstanding group of experienced leaders.

The distribution industry is filled with many talented entrepreneurs. Most of these individuals possess a strong characteristic that drives their success in building a network of business partners. Very seldom you might find an entrepreneur that embodies numerous characteristics which lend themselves to growing a business, a culture of love, respect, and virtue. Stormy Wellington is one that exemplifies these uncommon attributes in an industry filled with competitive personalities. The combination of faith, drive, and intelligence has propelled Stormy into the elite ranks of Executive Ambassador at TLC.

Stormy has refined her ability to mentor many business partners, while attracting hundreds at a time, on daily calls and live social media feeds. Stormy leads her prospects with tough love. If someone hesitates on their decision to purchase a product or join her movement, it'll most likely be the last time they speak with her. Successful entrepreneurs understand that business is a number's game. The more you reach, the more likely you will find success. Stormy has reached thousands on her way to becoming a top earner and now Executive Ambassador in TLC.

Her primary goal was to help 1,000 families earn over $100,000 dollars. Starting a new business venture is an exhilarating experience for many entrepreneurs. Stormy provides some insight into launching a business the right way. She explained that she remained extremely focused during the first 48 hours of joining TLC. She had a deep belief that she was going to regain the respect that she had lost.

She believes that money loves speed, and even though she didn't know everything about the TLC plan, she understood fast start bonuses and retail. She set two major goals for my first 30 days with the TLC. She was going to recruit 100 people and lose as much weight as I could using the products so she'll have a product testimony.

Stormy remains faithful and committed to her family, and friends. She understands that she has a greater purpose. She wants others to be inspired by her words and her actions. She has taken all her success and shared it with her family and friends. She enjoys being able to provide for them. Her ultimate mission was to help 1,000 families make

6 figures, but now she wants to help 1,000 families become millionaires.

Denise and William Lee are in the suburban part of Philadelphia, Pennsylvania. They recently reached the Ambassador rank in TLC. Each of them worked extremely hard to develop their careers. Their 24 year old son who currently lives in Los Angeles, is an entrepreneur who made the rank of executive director with TLC. Their daughter is also doing very well as an 18 year old model. Denise officially retired as a registered nurse and her next goal is to get her husband William to retire as well.

William and Denise Lee began promoting a schedule of opportunity calls every evening. Everyday the number of attendees grew larger and they became more comfortable delivering their message of helping others earn extra income. They didn't promise hundreds or thousands of dollars, or a bunch of dreams. Instead, they discussed how an extra $500-$1,000 per month could impact a family. Extra income helps to dissolve debt, and becomes the beginning of building residual income. William and Denise started to experience plenty of growth as a result of their opportunity calls. They decided to begin hosting weekend events in their hometown near Philadelphia to help distributors succeed.

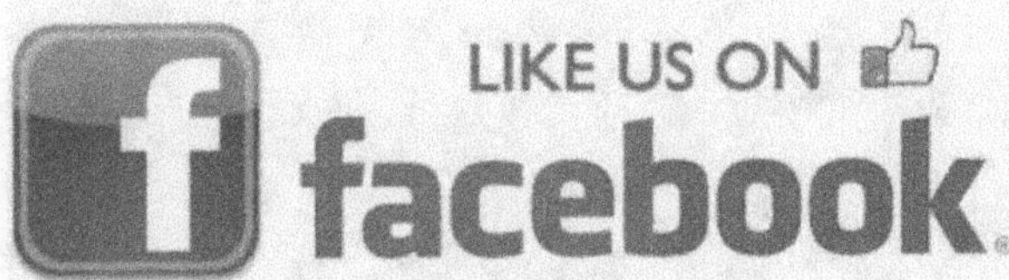

#LifeChangingReps

Find us on Google [Life Changing Reps] or in any search
browser.

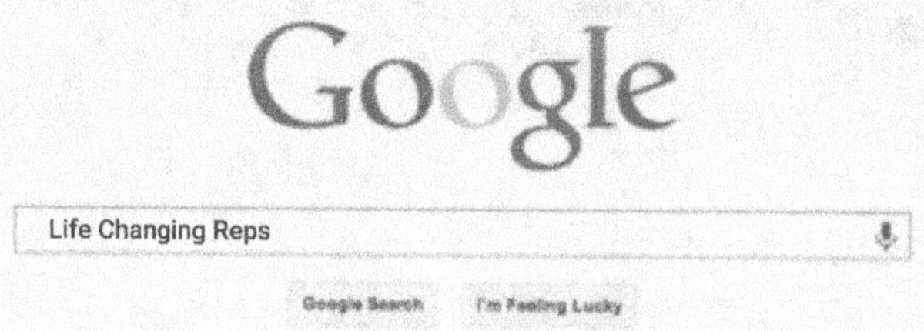

Subscribe to our channel for the latest updates on health and wellness products & services.

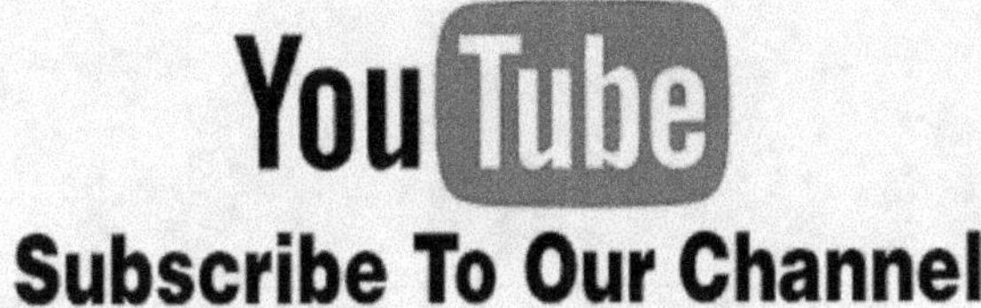

Terrell Barnes Life Changing Rep

TO: _______________________

FROM: _______________________

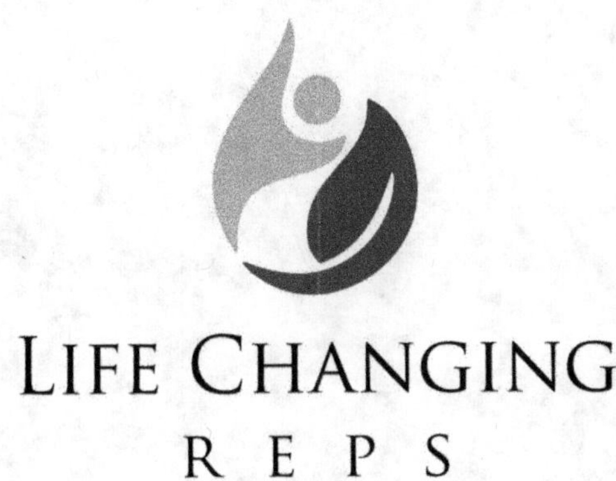